Practical Cruis

Seasickness

Paul Constantine

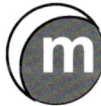

**Moonshine
Publications**

Seasickness

© Paul Constantine. 2012
Published & distributed in the UK by
Moonshine Publications,
Woodbridge, Suffolk
14 / IP12 4EU

ISBN 978-0-9572161-0-5

British Library Cataloguing in Publication Data.
A catalogue record for this book is available from the British Library.

Edited. Typeset & Design. Paul Constantine

Distributed. www.moonshinepublications.co.uk.

Printed. Bookwell OY. Teollisuustie 4, FI-06150, Porvoo. Finland.

DO NOT READ THIS BOOK

If you are you suffering from
seasickness at this moment

If so, it's **too late** to read this.
Reading can make you sick.
Do these things and read the rest later.

1. Have a bucket or a bowl in case you need it.
But try hard not to use it.

2. Lie down.
Wedged in a corner to stop you moving. Use no energy.
Fresh air is good, but you must not get cold.

3. Close your eyes.
Rest as much as you can.
Try to enjoy the rocking motion.
Relax.
Falling asleep is very good.

You can't do much more than this, so **stop reading**.
Go below and lie down

Seasickness

Only to be read when there is no chance of seasickness starting

This isn't a scientific/medical book

If you want to know about the detailed science of seasickness look it up on your computer in a search engine. Knowing only the science isn't really going to help you with the actual problem of dealing with seasickness when the time comes. You'll just be sick. What you really, really want to know is how to control it or deal with it when it strikes you … in a practical way. Understanding it and taking the right actions is what this book is aiming at. You may accept or reject it but I believe that if you try to understand how it works, you will feel more confident in working through it, as others before you have done.

With **understanding** you **CAN** make a big difference,

saving yourself a lot of discomfort.

Sufferers want to know:

What can I DO about seasickness?

That is where this might help.

1

Seasickness

Understanding

Ideally this needs to be read BEFORE you get yourself involved with seasickness so that you have some strategies to help you through it and help you to conquer it if you can. **But there are no guarantees of success;** *you have to see how it turns out for you. There is no single magic bullet, no wave of the wand. This is reality.*

Knowing enough to understand

If you do look up seasickness to find out what causes it you'll probably find that the medical experts say it is caused by the balance mechanism in your ears being upset by the movement. It is a bit of a surprise when you first learn this.

Seasickness is something to do with my ears!

It is hard to believe, but from this knowledge comes a difficult question that is rarely consciously asked:

If it is my **ears** *that are upset, why do I feel* **sick***?*

'Normal' sickness is something else, something to do with my stomach and what I've eaten, isn't it? Why am I **sick**? What is the link? Shouldn't I just feel dizzy or drunk or something to do with balance? **Why sick?** That doesn't make sense. Okay, those are good questions to ponder upon and they may lead us to a better understanding of what is happening. There have to be some good practical answers and it might be worth pursuing them, to discover where they might lead us. (*Incidentally, for the purpose of understanding, the sickness mechanism is nothing to do with your hearing, or the flappy things on either side of your head that we call 'ears', it's just that this is where the mechanism, technically called the* **vestibular system***, happens to be found in the body, so don't blame your actual ears.*) The sickness that lays us low is, however, connected with our bodies, and we are going to take a little time to look at how the body works, so please be patient. We are trying to keep this simple, trying to avoid technical words like 'vestibular' that we just used. We are just observing what happens, cause and effect. We are looking at ordinary, everyday happenings that we are familiar with, but maybe haven't thought about too deeply.

2

Understanding Cause and Effect.

Your (very clever) body

Your body operates on autopilot most of the time, but you've probably never really appreciated that. Your body has become so experienced at standing you up, sitting you down, changing from a walk to a run, going upstairs or down, or jumping, lying, rolling, spinning and any amount of other movements that your body is capable of, it just never bothers to tell you when it is handling the latest things that you have ordered it to do. It learned all this stuff years ago, right back at the beginning when you mastered crawling, shuffling, and then walking, step by unsteady step, with a leg at each corner, encouraged by your admiring relatives, and it has refined the skills over the intervening time, so that you now think that you are a master of movement. Clever you. You can do it without even thinking. Watch any toddler. They are programmed to learn this ultra-complex series of tasks, like standing up and walking about. Amazingly, in doing this they actually stand on one leg whilst moving. Even though each step involves coordinating some 200 muscles (*Dr Alice Roberts MB, BCh, BS, 'Origin of Us' television series*), it doesn't take them very long at all.

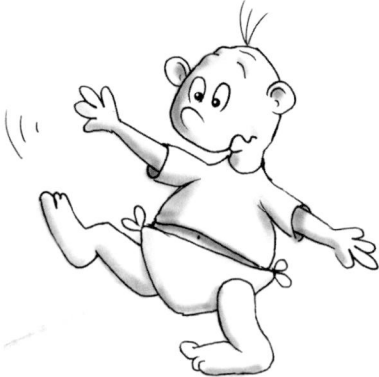

Now let us say that you move forward in years from being a toddler.

You are a teenager and you try to learn something new, a new kind of movement. Take up skiing or skateboarding. Learn to ride a surfboard or windsurfer and you will find yourself a toddler again, educating your body to accept this new kind of movement. You start with a lot of falling over and sitting down. As you learn, your body will impose an initial emotion of 'slight apprehension' upon you. This is a caution that makes you behave in a certain way. It slows you down to give the body the opportunity to absorb the new input relating to the new circumstances. The body can process this

3

information and relate it to what it already knows. It gradually becomes accustomed to it, understands it and stores it away so that when it meets the same set of circumstances again it can call upon the responses that it has already set by, for just such an input as this. If you master these skills you feel clever, because many other people do not. They give up. Why should they put themselves through this discomfort when they have no need to? They can manage without these 'more advanced' skills. This shows that learning new physical skills needs application, perseverance and practice.

Body or Brain?

I am calling it your body, but the bit that is being educated is, of course, based mainly inside your brain and it is this that is controlling your limbs to master the new circumstances. Remember learning to ride a bike? Watch a child doing this. Watch the parent running alongside offering advice and a steadying hand. The child's brain is receiving visual messages from what it sees, audible messages from what it is being told, sensory contact messages from the wind on the face, the feet on the pedals, the hands on the handlebars, complex muscle movement, the memory, having watched others do this, the knowledge that to fall at speed can hurt. The child is blending all this together and making the many adjustments required to achieve the desired result. It is so complex it is a wonder that it ever works, but it does, thanks to the super-computer that is the brain, your brain.

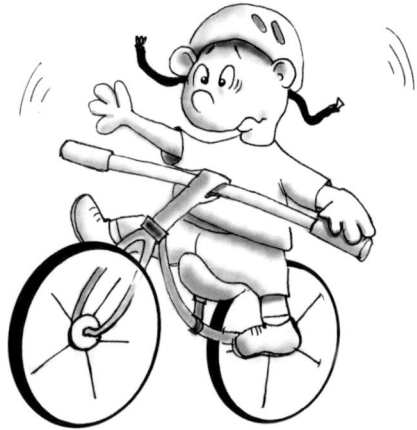

Move on again, to something a bit more extreme.

You want to learn to walk a tightrope. You are going rock climbing, parachuting or extreme bungee jumping. Now your body or brain will impose another emotion on you, fear. Real fear can have a

Seasickness

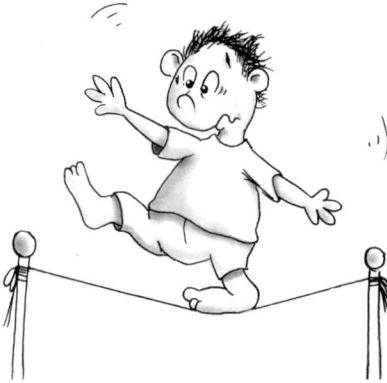

number of effects, but fundamentally, at first they add up to trying to stop you. The brain still receives all the outside stimuli, mainly from sight. The eyes see the edge of the precipice and the brain knows that this indicates danger, so it will immediately try to stop the body going further, whilst rapidly trying to prepare the body for what it perceives might come about. There may be a feeling of faintness. Some people go weak at the knees. The heartbeat may increase. To continue forward means overriding them, forcing them back.

These and other reactions are automatic responses that the body or brain selects and imposes. The subconscious part of your brain is sensing everything that you do and deciding which information should receive your conscious attention. The conscious part of your brain is limited to only about 2 or 3 tasks that can be handled at any one time, so it uses the power of the subconscious to filter and prioritise the input-deluge it is receiving.

The body/brain combination has a set of even more extreme responses to the next step of 'terror', but we have no need to go there. We can return to these observations about 'fear' later, but for now here is an important thought for you to evaluate that might help you later with fear:

Fear is almost always about the unknown.

Training

People do participate in challenging activities such as those already mentioned, and also in other extreme sports. They are able to do so because they usually go through some kind of training. The actions a person must take in extreme circumstances are explained to them and they are encouraged to learn the 'response-skills' piece by piece and then blend them together to master the appropriate actions. As they do this, the fear they may have experienced will slowly subside as the brain gains the knowledge to overcome the adversity. Once the unknown becomes known, participating in the challenging activity can even become pleasurable. Some people choose to jump out of aeroplanes or dive to the bottom of the sea without breathing equipment, but with such activities we have reached an even higher threshold and may think: *Why should I put myself through this discomfort when I have no need to? I can manage without these 'super-advanced' skills.* So most of us give them a miss. Very sensible.

Education and training can prepare the body for all manner of situations, circumstances and actions. The ordinary 'person in the street' appreciates watching trained people, athletes, sports people and entertainers demonstrating out-of-the-ordinary physical skills, be they trapeze artist, gymnast or ski-jumper. The public will pay to watch them, knowing that they do not have the skill or nerve to equal the person who has been specialist trained.

The Body/Brain combination

The point of all this is to appreciate that the body and brain work together in responding to external stimuli. They need training to become effective in new situations and they need to gain experience. They have their own way of operating, and although most people believe that they are always controlling their own body by sending it conscious commands, this is not always the absolute truth. In some cases the body/brain auto-response is the first to decide on appropriate action, and it IS capable of overriding the conscious thoughts of the person concerned.

This is the basic situation governing what is sometimes called 'motion sickness' and what we have also been calling 'seasickness'. We need to observe this even more closely now to understand exactly what is happening.

Motion Sickness

Whilst car sickness, air sickness and even 'space' sickness, together with seasickness, are all technically the same thing, described as 'motion sickness', there are added elements for seasickness that makes it much more difficult to deal with than just 'plain' motion sickness, as we will see later.

You can suffer motion sickness by riding in a car or going on a fairground ride. We can observe and learn several things from these experiences. First, is that different people have different levels of tolerance to the motion effect, but that the tolerance can be improved by experience (a kind of training).

In the days before most people had cars, when people did not travel long distances very frequently, motion sickness was more common when finally they did travel in a vehicle. Car travel is now commonplace, so most people have adjusted to the nature of the motion by the time they are no longer children. Science now tells us that we are born with about 100 billion neurons in our brains, and as we experience things a series of links is formed between them. The connections are called dendrites and they allow the brain cells to 'talk' to each other.

If you never experience an event, the connections are never made.

The more times an event is experienced the thicker the connections become. If the experiences are reduced, the connections are cut back to make the brain more efficient. Knowing this allows us to see that if we get the experience of being on the sea when we are young, the connections will be forged. If we don't go afloat for many years afterwards then the connections will need 'refreshing', depending on how long it was since we had the last experience. It's another case of 'use it or lose it'. It is also the case that the connections CAN be made, but it takes time, and generally speaking, as with most learning, 'the older you are, the slower', depending upon what other related experiences a person has had. A child that learned to skateboard early will probably move more easily onto a windsurfer, then onto a surfboard, then skis or a snowboard followed by ice skates, than one that has never honed their 'balance' skills in any way. This is why it is essential for us to learn a language and to read, write, make mathematical calculations and learn to play a musical instrument, amongst other things, early in life, in order to lay down the network of neuron connections (called a neural network) in our brains when we are young. The experience of going to sea on a smallish boat, whilst still young, is one that has escaped most people in our modern days. When it does happen, the brain has nothing in its networks to even make a start with, and it can be an extreme learning experience. In most cases the brain has to begin from a zero position and (it is worth repeating) it will take TIME.

An experienced but susceptible person's system might still be caught out by the extremes of a fairground ride, and we also sometimes see television reporters looking distinctly green after being 'fortunate' enough to be taken for a ride in an aerobatic aeroplane. This shows that there may be a reasonable tolerance to 'average' motion sickness within the general population, but taking someone beyond their normal levels of motion can trigger an 'overload' reaction. Here comes another relevant question.

How does the body know that it is experiencing unusual movements?

The answer has already been mentioned. The brain gets messages from **sight**, **sound** and **sensory contact** input. It is worth looking at these in yet more detail, because their effects are very powerful, more powerful than might be expected.

Sight alone is the single most powerful input, and here is an interesting example. A television series about 'Towns' looked at waste disposal systems and the way that rubbish is tipped onto a moving conveyor belt for sorting. Operatives picked off certain categories of rubbish such as cardboard etc. The presenter Nick Crane was told that it is difficult to find people capable of enduring this task, because most will suffer from motion sickness. Some can manage a few weeks, some less than an hour. Indeed, when he tried it, he too experienced feeling queasy within a very short time.

Motion sickness … without body motion?

How can this be? Although an operator was standing normally it was the unusual circumstance of the constant movement of the conveyor belt filling the field of vision that tricked the brain into trying to calculate how to respond to what it took to be bodily movement. Finding no tried and proven responses in its memory banks to apply to such a situation, it triggered its automatic response. Sickness. It is possible to experience a similar effect from playing racing games on a computer. This kind of motion sickness, where the body is stationary, upright or seated, but with incoming overwhelming messages indicating that there is movement, is almost the opposite to seasickness, where there is violent external movement. In a car the eyes can say that the body is travelling at speed, but the body (the vestibular system in the ears) can say that it is seated and at rest at the very same time. This is the confusing mismatch of information that the brain must try to resolve. Irrespective of the mode of travel or the situation, the body's response is exactly the same, almost instant 'overload' and a demand (through sickness) for the situation to STOP until a solution can be generated. If 'sound' and 'sensory' messages reinforce what 'sight' is saying to the brain, then the effect can be almost total and not to be questioned. So complete are these three monitoring systems that if we can trick them we can be entertained by the effect.

In France there is a huge theme park called 'Futuroscope' near Poitier. In a series of futuristic pavilions customers can go and watch a variety of short films. Whilst each film is a bit different, they all seek to enhance the 'normal' film experience. Many are 3D, thus giving depth to the on-screen image. Most have huge screens that fill the field of vision right to the very edges, unlike a normal cinema screen. Some have wrap-around screens to reduce distortion at the edges of the field of vision. Then there are the seats that the audience is sitting on. Some seats are synchronised to move with the moving screen image. The movement is not great, just a little up and down or tipping from side to side. As the 3D image takes you on a fairground ride the glasses you wear sometimes have tiny speakers relaying surround-sound directly into your ears, you sway from side to side on those special seats as you corner and maybe a hidden nozzle in the back of the seat in front blows air into your face. The affect is total. It is real. It is not that you are *imagining* flying across the Grand Canyon or skiing down a mountain, you actually ARE, because there is no sight, sound or sensory contact information that indicates anything to the contrary. It is so real that you have to be strapped into your seat before it begins, so real that on some rides you may have your hands on a steering device to try to give you some feeling of control. You 'lose your tummy' over the bumps, you sweat when you look down at the void beneath you and your hands grip tightly to stop your fall. Some of the most effective rides can take you into different worlds, flying over amazing landscapes and through superb surroundings. What you see and feel IS where you are. Sometimes it can be scary enough to make you close your eyes. You can shout with fear, you duck or hold up your hands to protect yourself. *(Look along the rows of seats and see everyone reacting in the same evasive way, in unison.)* When the film ends and the lights go on, to gasps of relief, everyone will have the biggest smile of enjoyment and of amazement at the realisation that they could have been so comprehensively transported away, whilst simply sitting in a chair in a darkened room.

Something similar happens in flight simulators, and fairgrounds have used similar tricks in the past. One funfair trick is very relevant here. Put several people into a room that has images of all the normal doors, windows and furnishings projected onto the walls that surround them. You can imagine these walls as an inverted box suspended over the people, but they don't know that. They only see that they are in a 'normal' room. They stand and look around at their normal surroundings. Now suddenly, sharply, tip to one side the suspended box that is their walls. All the people will fall over, even though the ground they are standing on remains quite steady. They fall because at the instant they perceived the room to move, they made an immediate compensating move of the body in the opposite direction to remain standing upright. The image that the eyes were relaying to the brain took all its visual cues from the upright edges of doors, corners, windows and pictures etc.

The brain knows what is upright as it monitors these visual cues at all times when the eyes are open. It is hardwired to do this because the process was learned so early and it has never been challenged over all the intervening years. The brain's stored 'movement-memory' did need refining a bit for travelling on motor vehicles, or trains or planes, but it has rarely been challenged quite as severely as when the brain is totally caught out by the funfair trick. If this happens only once then the brain may discard it as an infrequent event of only minor importance, not needing storage for later, but if the brain is taken not to the funfair, but out to sea, then that will be quite a different circumstance as it will be a much longer, more continuous event. Going on the sea is a serious environmental change needing some serious brain reprogramming.

So now, with the benefit of what we have observed,
we can return to the question posed much earlier.
Why am I SICK?

Why am I sick?

Think of it like this. We have already mentioned that on land, in the home, the eyes look outwards and see images that are familiar, of items and objects that they know to be upright; doorframes are a good example. From a stream of observed cues the brain can keep the body in an upright stance and feel secure that it has things under its control. It has done this for years. However, when on the sea, the brain begins by casually processing this same stream of commonly observed details only to suddenly find that the doorframe is not upright. This is something that has never happened before. It searches for confirmation or alternatives in the incoming information and finds nothing of any real use that can be quickly referenced to correct the basic bank of knowledge. The only real reference at sea is the horizon, which remains constantly *horizontal*. If the body is down below on a boat, the horizon cannot be seen, it cannot be used, but 'inexperienced' brains do not usually have even this knowledge anyway. This is the fairground trick of being in the moving room, but it is not just a single movement that has to be processed; it is a constant stream of movements back/forth and up/down. Subtle forces on muscles, such as acceleration, gravity and inertia, are in conflict with sight, sound and sensory contact.

There are structures in the balance mechanism that tell the brain when the head is moving in a straight line and also indicate the position of the head in relation to the pull of gravity. Difficulties occur when the left and right balance systems are not working together, so the brain thinks the head is moving when it is not. If the head is moved in opposition to what other sensory messages are saying, the situation becomes even worse. The brain will be utterly confused, but it isn't just a question of 'What is upright?' that is the total problem.

The added demands of visual micromovement

Worse than this, below deck in a moving boat, something else very strange is also going on. This is happening at a subconscious level beyond rational control. Normally, on land, whenever you put out your hand to pick up something the brain is doing some lightning calculations about the position of the object, the direction of travel of the hand, how far the hand has to go and where it has to arrive to successfully contact the chosen article. When the hand arrives, it naturally picks up the article. However, at sea, this 'automatic' function is no longer operating accurately. The hand reaches for the doorframe to steady the body, but the doorframe has moved from the place that it was in when the hand started on its journey. A swift recalculation is required at the last moment to make a successful contact between hand and doorframe. This means uprating the processing speed of the brain. Everything that the eyes are looking at is moving minutely, everything needs checking and re-checking. This micromovement generates a kind of visual blur not consciously seen. The brain must go faster in a situation where other things are also going from bad to worse. The whole body has to sway constantly, seeking an unknown vertical, muscles have to be braced first one way and then another to counteract the surging and constant movement that is going on.

The sense of balance doesn't rely entirely on visual input. It also uses an awareness of key body parts relative to the place that the body is in, its surroundings. The brain has to know where the feet and legs are in relation to the upper body. It learns this from movement detectors in the muscles, tendons and joints, particularly in the ankles, legs and hips compared to the neck. By constantly monitoring the relative positions it prioritises the messages according to circumstances. It will give extra credibility to muscular information if the eyes cannot see, thus allowing the body to remain standing even in a pitch dark room. I have sailed with a totally blind sailor who was completely able to run his own boat due to his vast experience. He operated without any visual input. For the inexperienced, the confusing sounds are all new and of limited help, but still need processing. The ground (trustworthy until now) cannot be used as a reference. What is happening? The brain is racing and cannot keep up. It is overloading. It wants it all to slow down (as in apprehension); it wants it all to stop (as in fear). It is getting an overload of information, and this must cease until reprogramming can take place. The brain MUST play an ace card to make the body STOP (*make it lie down*); it must STOP the incoming information by halting the confusing, mainly visual input (*closing the eyes*). The body is told to feel sick (*overriding any conscious wishes*) by central brain command and, generally speaking, this has the desired effect. You do not have to close your eyes when you lie down, but if you are so weakened and lacking in energy (the immediate effects) due to sickness, you WILL close your eyes.

The brain has now achieved, by automatic reflex, the two most important pieces of advice that we started with at the beginning of this book:

1. Lie down. 2. Close your eyes.

Seasickness
What happens now?

This is how to think of it. The rest time given to the brain allows it to backtrack to basics and start rewriting some of the assumptions that it has always held. Parts of the brain that were suffering from information-overload can be cleared and retrieved for further processing as part of the recovery process that is about to take place. This takes time. The overload was partially caused by the visual micromovement, the general reprogramming for 'upright' and 'muscle memory' together with the 'total learning' required by the new environmental demands of the uniquely special surroundings of being in a randomly moving capsule. The brain begins to deal with the information, or data overload.

Information-overload

Information-overload is a kind of mental fatigue that can be experienced when the brain is trying to process an unusually large amount of input in a sustained way. It gets no rest and has to go on and on processing rapidly, assessing, cross-referencing and making decisions based on information that perhaps has not been fully evaluated. Strategies for dealing with information-overload are mentioned later, including the especially important **'snapshotting'**.

It is possible to feel the beginnings of information-overload separately from seasickness. For example, in your car you try to find your way to a strange street, in a strange town, without using your Satnav. You only know the street's approximate location and you have never seen the busy, traffic-filled roads that you are driving on before. In addition to monitoring all driving controls, now being taken over almost totally by your inbuilt automatic driving pilot (*car-driving section of the brain*) that has been specialist-trained for this purpose, you have to watch all external traffic movements (for the safety of your vehicle and the body inside it). This is the most taxing demand. Additionally, you must read the road signs all around you and make snap judgements about what actions to take, which lane, when to turn, when to stop. You will automatically slow down, to

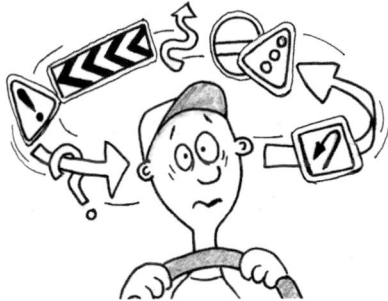

13

limit the inflow of information, to give the brain more time. Other, local drivers whiz past, cursing your ineptitude and spotting you as a hazard long before you see them coming, as you hardly have time to use your rear-view mirrors. If you continue too long at this test you may get a slight whirling dizziness. Continue further and you may experience momentary vagueness of thought, little gaps where you think you missed something. This can develop, as can that almost dizzy feeling, followed by a realisation that you will have to stop to check the map, ask someone, or just reassess the whole situation before you end up driving the wrong way up a one-way street. These sensations of information-overload are not to be recommended in cars, and the following circumstances are to be avoided at all cost, but they are important to look at and evaluate.

Some other related observations here. People will tell you that travelling is tiring. On a long car journey it is generally true that the car's driver can stay awake for much longer than the passengers, despite having the greater responsibility and having to process much more information. Car passengers, having no responsibility, watch the road and the passing scenery, which produces a great deal of information to be processed. The information may be of little practical use, but it is mildly interesting. The brain will filter it and absorb a proportion, but when it reaches a reasonable capacity it allows the process to stop by closing the eyes to reduce input. This is the natural response to approaching overload, and the brain will clear the backlog through sleep, ready to begin again.

The passenger does not have a 'responsibility for safety' trigger to counteract this process, as the driver does. So the passengers usually fall asleep before the driver, entrusting their safety to the driver. Adult car passengers can remain fresher, longer (preparing to take over the driving before the driver gets too tired) by simply closing their eyes (looking as though they are asleep). This greatly reduces the visual information they have to process, bringing it right down to a minimum.

The driver on the other hand has responsibility for the safety of all. It is this knowledge that initially keeps him/her awake, but it is this that carries the driver beyond the normal, natural limits of information input. However, there is a limit to everything and the driver cannot go on for ever. If the driver continues for too long he or she will begin to suffer information-overload made worse by physical muscular fatigue, characterised by short patches of blank consciousness, where effectively the brain is briefly switching off.

The blanks are a form of sleep even if the eyes are open. The brain is trying to find some space, some interruption in the constant information input. This is very dangerous. If the driver persists, the blanks will get longer as the brain gets to a point where it just cannot take in any more. The driver becomes drowsy. Eventually the eyes will close. Vehicles do not fail 'safe' and this kind of thing can result in fatalities. This is why there are sensible time limits recommended for drivers, to encourage them to rest.

Some of these driving situations can also be related to sailing. One of the ways to help stave off seasickness on yachts is to allow a person in the early stages of feeling queasy to do some steering. This diverts and engages the brain. It gives them the 'driver's responsibilities', but it may not be a 'cure', as it will gradually add to their fatigue. More of this a little later.

The recovering brain

The brain recovers best from information-overload during proper sleep. Cutting-edge scientists may explain that it is all to do with connecting your 100 billion neurons with dendrites in a neural network, but let's keep a simple image in our minds. Let's say that in general terms the brain filters, re-orders and re-stores the material it has in its 'To-Do' tray, putting it into appropriate filing-cabinet categories of associated information (*giving rise to dreams as some memories are reshuffled to make way for the new ones*). When all this is tidy there is the space to process the new stuff it has to deal with, for us, this mainly concerns movement or motion.

Responses to motion

The main problem for the brain seems to be the thousands of readjustments that have to be made due to the tiny movements it perceives in 'normal' processes. This is what we called 'visual micromovement'. It is worth reminding ourselves about this. Let us take reading as an example.

Your eyes can be directed to these static words on the page with ease and the proper focus 'dialled' into your pupils, retina etc. as a single operation right at the beginning of the reading process. The book stays where it is. The head stays where it is. The muscles controlling arm, hand, neck and head, finger grip pressure holding the book, all stay more or less the same. Now try it whilst you are sailing. If the whole world starts moving, the body needs bracing and the book is making oscillating movements from side to side whilst going back and forth, no matter how slightly, then the amount of information to be processed expands exponentially. For this reason, on boats, as we said right at the beginning:

Reading can make you sick
(as does any concentrated visual activity)

Any 'small' activity requiring the coordination of hand and eye can do this. On board, you may not be doing jigsaw puzzles or knitting, which would have a similar effect, but you could be doing mathematical calculations relating to tide and time, speed and distance sailed, entering waypoints or recording the log. You should be aware that these might be heavy on the mental/physical information to be processed. Okay, so these mental gymnastics are not reading, but the processing, the hand/eye coordination is almost the same, and it is this that is causing the trouble. We can also now add awareness of several other conditions that are going to affect susceptibility to seasickness.

Let us look at a few more factors that could add to the possibility of bringing on seasickness, to make you fully aware of them and allow you to counteract them if necessary by modifying what you do.

Smells can make you feel sick

The worst of these is the distinctive smell of sickness itself. If someone else is being sick, try to stay upwind of them. This is good advice anyway as they should be to leeward in a boat's cockpit and secured so that they cannot fall out in their weakened state. Being sick to windward is a guarantee of 'getting your own back'. If people are being sick inside boats it is worth helping them by emptying their bowl/bucket and rinsing it for them at the appropriate moment … if you can. A half-mug of fresh water to rinse their mouth will always be appreciated. Such assistance will also help you, by keeping the air smelling sweeter down below.

If you are on a passenger ship it may be much more difficult to avoid the smell, particularly in certain areas, such as toilets. Stepping out onto a sheltered deck (well wrapped up against the cold) has to be considered preferable to remaining below if the smell begins to be a problem.

Most people don't like the smell of diesel in confined spaces, so having to work on an engine is not to be recommended, especially as visual micromovement will be added to your problems if you are engaged in intense hand/eye coordination with your head upside-down in the bilge.

Some people just cannot tolerate cooking smells, especially the frying of fatty food, but if the sea is rough enough most crew, with no matter how much experience, will be dissuaded from cooking a full English breakfast, simply because of the difficulty in securing all the components required, in the pan, on the stove.

Fatigue can make you sick

If bad weather persists on a voyage and the skipper or crew are working long hours getting little rest, they will begin to experience the symptoms of information-overload, leading eventually to 'blank patches' and then a gradual inability to make meaningful decisions or undertake straightforward calculations. Such conditions bring on, or prolong, the conditions for seasickness. Very tired people can appear to be in a state of waking sleep, which they probably are.

It is tiring just being on a boat in a seaway. If you are wearing full sea kit of harness, lifejacket, oilskin top, oilskin trousers and boots over your warm clothes, it is hard, hard work going below to use the toilet. The process of getting undressed, using the facility and then getting dressed again can easily take half an hour or more and it is an exhausting process.

Fear can make you sick

Many sailors don't like to admit this, but it is true. The more macho they are, the harder it is to admit. We have looked at fear before and it is worth repeating this: Fear is almost always about the unknown. If you are new to sailing and do not know what to expect, then you may experience fear early, if conditions are poor.

There are ways to combat fear. The first step is to identify this is a factor in what is causing the problem and then **admit it** to yourself. It is particularly hard if you are the skipper. If you can say to yourself, 'What am I scared of?' you will usually find that the roughness of the seas and the wind noise are the immediate causes. The noise can be overpowering and the motion tremendous, but these alone probably do not threaten your safety whilst your boat remains able. It is your boat and its equipment that will save you, and so you must have faith in them. Before you even departed you needed to have **total** faith in the boat, its equipment and very importantly, the *experience of the person in charge.* This is a quote from Thomas Firth Jones' book *Multihull Voyaging* published by Sheridan House: *'The essence of multihull voyaging is to trust your vessel after making sure that it is a vessel you can trust. The trustworthiness is in the design and seamanship.'* It applies equally to all monohulls. There have been notable disasters in offshore yacht races such as the Fastnet or the Sydney Hobart that have generated much information about extreme weather conditions and people's reactions to horrifying situations. Things can happen aboard any boat that may suddenly bring fear even to the most experienced sailors. A friend told me of an incident when he was crewing a yacht across the North Sea. The conditions weren't comfortable, the boat was being thrown about, but all on board were seasoned sailors and they were pushing on, so they were about 30 miles offshore. Cockpit conversations drifted down to the skipper and off-watch crew resting below. There was a note of concern. The man on the helm was having trouble steering the yacht; the listeners paid attention. Then he said, 'It feels like the rudder has dropped off.' Immediately, those below were dragging on oily jackets and exiting the companionway into the wilder weather conditions on deck. They were all gathering, trying to rapidly assess the situation, when without word, without warning, the owner/skipper violently threw up the contents of his stomach across the back of my friend and into the rest of the cockpit. He was a very experienced man. This wasn't motion sickness, it was sickness at sea. We can guess that it was more likely to be the instant weight of responsibility and the fleeting subconscious thought that the integrity of the craft that they all relied upon was compromised. In no time at all they had moved from 'normal' to 'life threatening' for the crew and the boat, and one man took that responsibility upon himself. Further investigation showed that it was the rudder steering linkage that had failed, and they made it back safely using the emergency steering kit. A few buckets of seawater cleared up the mess. This was an extreme and unusual circumstance, but it does illustrate how fear can be a contributory factor to the complex condition that we are exploring.

One thought that it is important to hold onto is that the boat can usually survive better than the crew. Fear is in the mind, and the more powerful the imagination, the greater the fear of what might happen. Generally, it is true that people are thinking to themselves, 'what **might** happen?' If it hasn't already happened, try to stay calm. It is usually the **threat** of the waves, and this implies that it has not yet happened. You are worrying about the 'unknown' that might come after the event, without actually visualising what actions you would take at that time. There is sometimes this 'vagueness' in fear. Take all reasonable steps to ensure your safety. Be mentally prepared. Make sure that you have done all that you can do and that you are ready, and then rest as much as you can. You can do no more. Statistically speaking, loss of life at sea from yachts is very rare, and sadly more people are drowned in garden pools or ponds than lose their lives on yachts at sea. More people are drowned in cars running off roads into water, than in boats, so take heart. If it hasn't happened yet, start to think it **might not** happen. Be as prepared as you can be, but think positively.

Fear has to be admitted, analysed and responded to logically, in order to gain control over it. It may then subside slightly.

Fear for the less experienced

Suppose you find yourself in a scary sea state and you are frightened of the waves. One little trick to try, if possible (ensuring that you are well enough and well secured) is to attempt to get a photograph of an exceptionally big and threatening wave as it approaches. If you get it, you can use it to amaze your friends back on land and it will prove just how bad the conditions were that you endured. Most people find themselves waiting with the camera at the ready, waiting, waiting, and waiting. 'Here comes one! ... No, not big enough; here's another ... no, we've had bigger than that.' After some time the thought begins to intrude that maybe the sea isn't quite as bad as you thought, now that you are getting used to it. If you do get a snap, take a look at it. Is it terrifying?

    I am not trying to belittle what is happening to you, but I am saying that through being new to an experience the body/brain will perceive it with some apprehension, maybe fear, and finally perhaps terror in extremely rare circumstances. Each person has to build up a yardstick against which to measure that experience. If you are new to the game you will look to your more experienced companions and monitor their reactions. If they remain controlled, then you should take courage from that. 'They in their turn will have their own fear thresholds. They may be thinking, This isn't as bad as that time when we were … Or, another time when …' Experience lifts the limit-levels where acceptance changes to apprehension, or then changes into fear, and, as mentioned much earlier, training and knowing what to expect will help you to get a grip on it.

It is true that fear is fatiguing. You may find that all your muscles are held tensed up. You have to tell them to relax. If you are not actively engaged in running the ship, lie down, wedged in, eyes closed. Take away the noise by listening to music or a radio through earphones. You can be mentally transported away for a time by a studio discussion, by a tennis match, by an entertainer or a story, and you will be more relaxed whilst you do this, conserving energy ready for when it is really needed.

Not using the toilet can contribute to making you feel sick

Now this is a strange thing to read. This is stuff that you do not normally consider when you think that you will go sailing on a yacht, so it's a bit of a surprise. It does need to be discussed, however, so that the inexperienced offshore sailor can understand what is likely

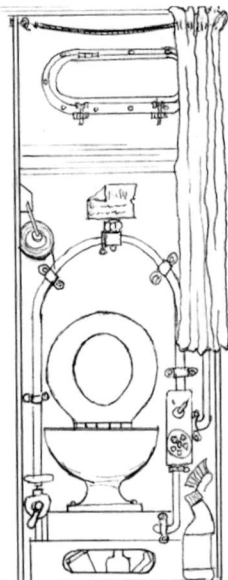

to happen and can be ready to combat it if/when it does.

When we eat food it should go through a natural process inside the body and come out of the other end. It is not meant to return via the route that it was put in, namely, your mouth. It is a great help if it keeps going through and doesn't get stuck, but sometimes it can. It is an unusual thing to assert, but most people have their own favourite toilet, in their own favourite bathroom, at home. They hardly think about its use that is automatic. Put them into the typically constricted thin-walled box aboard a boat that is called the toilet (or 'heads'), with its strange array of valves, levers, handles or buttons, and it is not as easy to relax as it is at home. Is it too politically incorrect to say that women find this much more of an issue than men? The toilet, the cleanliness of it surroundings, the smell in its immediate area and the sounds generated when using it, are all of primary importance.

It is well known to the experienced sailor that marine toilets that have been unused for a few days will produce a sulphurous smell from the stagnant de-oxygenated water trapped in the pipes until they have been pumped through thoroughly. This is not good news for the inexperienced sailor meeting the situation for the first time. It is not helped by the prominent labels on the hardware, forbidding the use of bleaches and disinfectants (to preserve the valves). The apprehension associated with pumping pumps and opening and closing valves in the correct order for fear of sinking the boat, or clogging the system and possibly having to call the rest of the crew to unblock the pipes, is quite sufficient to produce a blockage inside the new sailor, rather than in the toilet pipes. What can begin as a mental block may develop into a physical one. Putting food in at the top end **must** result in food coming out at the bottom end to rejoin the food cycle. Preferably this should happen by the second day of sea sailing or else it could begin to become a contributory sickness problem. If all the food has already returned via the top end then there will be reduced need for it to exit properly, but that ability has to be restored as soon as possible.

It can be seen that familiarity with all these toilet factors can come with experience, and then they will be lower mental hurdles to be surmounted, but for the beginner it can all be yet another shock to the system, demanding adjustments by the brain to a new set of hygiene standards that weren't really expected. An early conscious decision has to be made to 'love the loo' that you are with, so as to keep the food flowing in the correct direction. Don't give the body the smallest excuse for not doing this. Using the toilet correctly is a sure sign that the body is adjusting to the challenge of the unusual motion, and is heading in the right direction.

A combination of factors increases the risk of seasickness

Whilst the scientific-medical explanations will concentrate mainly on the balance mechanism that just happens to be located inside your ears, we can now see that in total, it may be a bit more complicated.

A newcomer to the experience will begin to feel queasy from the main factors of the motion, but must also try to identify if there are additional contributory factors that can also be addressed. Ask yourself: Am I tired? Am I frightened? Am I smelling unpleasant

Seasickness

smells? Is there anything else? You can then take any extra precautions to minimise these other factors. There are other steps to take, but first we should look at the sickness process, always seeking to understand what is happening.

A very useful thing to know is how we are made to feel sick. Apparently the vomiting centre in the brain is stimulated by:
- the digestive tract
- thoughts and emotions
- the inner ear controlling balance
- receptors responding to harmful substances in the blood

If we set aside the last one, it will be seen that we can address positive actions, ourselves, to suppress or control the first three. It is interesting to see that 'thoughts and emotions' have an important contribution to offer (see *Sea legs,* later).

The Sickness Process

With the understandings that we might have gained, simply by observing the processes at work we can now formulate some ways of minimising the worst of the seasickness-inducing factors. There are different external circumstances that can affect the person about to suffer from seasickness according to their situation:

- on a ferry or cruise ship
- taking up employment at sea
- going to sail on a yacht at sea
- for a short journey or for an extended journey

You will appreciate how each of these situations differs from the others, but for each individual they have this question in common:

How will I be affected by seasickness?

If you are inexperienced, you don't know how you might be affected, and the effects have a very wide spectrum. Some people do not seem to be greatly affected, and on a short journey with a calm crossing perhaps the majority may experience no ill effects at all. The bigger the ship, the smaller the movement. Modern ships have stabilisers to damp down the movement. It is all very enjoyable and interesting and you'll wonder what all the fuss was about. Easy. Conclusion, I don't suffer from seasickness. Hooray!

At the opposite end of the scale is the young person who may be trying out commercial fishing and stepping onto the cold steel deck on a dark night to go to sea in February, to work hard for long hours surrounded by the smell of diesel and gutted fish. Yes, this is extreme and not within the compass of this book, except to say that hopefully it doesn't happen too often these days, and if it should, then the person concerned will have already had training and previous experience to build upon, to ready the body for the extremes of what is to come.

Reactions to sickness

On sailing yachts much will depend upon how individuals react to being sick. Obviously the act of being sick is not pleasant, but then what follows will probably be the divide between those who CAN go forward making progress through the experience to conquer their sickness and those who cannot. There are different grades of response to being seasick. Generally, this is what might happen.

After their first bout of sickness some people say 'Oh I feel much better now.' And they can then continue with what they were doing. They sometimes do not appreciate that this may not be the end of the process, and they may well be sick again after another 10 to 15 minutes, and then again, and then again at various intervals. They may still feel themselves to be a little better after each bout, but gradually their energy levels drop, as you might expect, until they begin to feel much weaker and then they just want to sit still and recover.

This is a typical process, and from observation I would say that they will probably recover and will eventually be okay, maybe within a day, maybe a couple of days, depending upon the length and roughness of the passage and the actions they take.

Then there are those who do not seem to recover. Being ill makes them tired beyond measure and they are constantly sick and exhausted, so that after three or four days they are still not eating and their best friend is their bucket, from which they cannot be parted. They lack energy, need to sleep a lot, have little to say and can only dream of this coming to an end as their heads loll about with every heave and surge of the boat. Once ashore they will probably opt not to put themselves through this experience, of 'prayer and fasting' as Mike Peyton calls it, again. They will know that sea sailing is not for them. It may be that they were unlucky with the sea conditions or the weather. It may be that with a longer time to acclimatise they could have made the transition, some people take a fortnight. But everyone will make up their own minds. Some will stick with it, and others may head for the golf course and prefer to use the Channel Tunnel in future.

They are not the worst sufferers. Some people become comatose. They can be hardly identifiable bundles of clothing in the corner of a cockpit floor, or they lie inert on their bunks and cannot be raised. They began the sickness process and then disappeared. The other crew sometimes discuss them, wonder about them, try to wake them, but it is to no avail. Gradually concern for them grows and eventually, if it is possible, the boat is diverted towards land where a doctor might be found. I have been on such journeys when as the boat was approaching the harbour wall, in still water at last, with lines and fenders rigged, a ghostly wraith, to the crew's amazement, appears at the companionway enquiring, 'Are we there then?' in a weak and wobbly voice. We thought they had died, but the cure was swift. It is said of seasickness that the one certain cure is to 'sit under a tree'. It is also said that *at first you fear that you might die, but eventually you fear that might **not** die!* Rest assured that for the vast majority it does not get this bad. My comatose companions have usually had nothing worse than a missing period in their lives, of which they have no recollection, as they stride up the street to the station with a spring in their step.

Short journeys or passengers on cruise ships and ferries

These are usually trips of limited duration. Probably the best advice is to avoid immediately heading for the bar to drink large quantities of alcohol. Generally, however, anyone apprehensive about such a voyage will usually be directed toward drugs or alternative treatments.

Drugs

Look them up on websites by entering 'seasickness', or go into the local chemist's shop and read the instructions on the boxes. It is a wise precaution to always check the dosage of seasickness or travel pills, as they can change from country to country. There is a lot of difference between a dose of 15 mg and one of 75 mg from similar-looking pills. You have to do this for yourself. **I cannot offer to advise you here,** but I can make some observations.

The drugs have different trade names according to which country they are in, but most of them try to tackle the symptoms by slowing down the body's reaction time to any stimuli. This is usually described as 'a mild sedative effect' or even 'a mild depressant effect on the brain'. Telling you the names of some of the many chemicals involved, such as, dimenhydrinate, cyclizine, hyoscine or cinnarizines isn't really going to help you and might make you sick by just reading them, but go ahead and research them if you wish.

The advice in the packet may tell you that the drug is an **antihistamine**, but does that take you any closer to an understanding? If you research this word you are more likely to get information that you do understand, rather than the individual names of the specific chemicals. You will discover that different

25

antihistamine drugs in different strengths, with different durations of action, are used to target a range of different ailments, usually concentrating on allergy reactions such as hay fever or insect bites and stings, but you can guess that this probably does not immediately relate to what we are directly concerned with here. You have to find your way through the maze by yourself selecting what is relevant and what is not.

It will tell you not to mix this drug with any others, especially alcohol, and we can understand that, because two drugs together, both with a relaxing effect, might just send the user off to sleep. It will warn you to seek medical advice if you are pregnant, have a heart condition or a list of other ailments that would make you cautious anyway about taking any drugs.

Another word to follow up on, if you wish, is **antiemetic,** which covers drugs that combat the feeling of nausea. The descriptions for the use of these drugs will include sickness due to pregnancy or having swallowed a harmful substance, so once again you have to extract what you feel is relevant to the special interest of seasickness. This might include information about labyrinthitis (probably caused by a viral infection of the inner ear) or vertigo (a spinning sensation), which both affect the balance mechanism in the ear. The same warnings about drowsiness will be offered for an antiemetic as for antihistamines, especially to be careful about driving or operating machinery.

An allied search of passing interest at this point is to put **electrolyte imbalance** into the search engine. This will explain how everybody has small quantities of many chemicals in the bloodstream that are known as 'electrolytes', such as calcium, magnesium, sodium, potassium. When they are dissolved in water they separate into negatively and positively charged ions. Nerve and muscle functions depend upon the exchange of these ions inside and outside body cells. The relevance of this to us is that prolonged periods of sickness can deplete the body of these substances, leading to an imbalance. Basically, this isn't good, and the levels need to be restored to normal by eating again. To say more than this will take us into a series of biochemical lectures, so it is up to you to research it, if it is important to you.

You will soon see that the drug companies are as concerned about travel sickness on land as they are about sickness at sea, because their customers will cover the complete range of transport. If they offer any additional advice specifically about seasickness it will probably be to stay on deck and look at the horizon, keeping away from diesel smells and fatty food.

We discovered that the brain was overloading itself with excessive information as it tried to deal with every little change it perceived in body movement or activity. Well, we can think that the action of some drugs is aimed at slowing down this rapid brain activity until it can adjust to the new circumstances. With the drugs the brain is not as sharply agile; it is downgrading a percentage of what is coming in. I think of it as maybe like looking at a scene through slightly frosted glass. The general image can be made out and understood, but the sharp edges of every object within the field of vision do not have to be precisely positioned and visually tracked. I am not saying that it stops the eyes from seeing. I am attempting to contrast the amount of information having to be processed within the two situations. The brain is learning to ignore unwanted signals, just as it does with the ticking of a clock in a quiet room, or the constant roar of traffic on a busy road outside the door.

There are warnings about 'drowsiness' on the packets, with advice not to drive. Most drugs are in pill form (some are in patches containing *scopolamine* to stick on the skin), and they have to be taken at least two hours before the time of exposure to seasickness conditions. Trying to take pills whilst in the process of sickness simply means that they get rejected like the rest of the stomach contents, so it's a waste of money trying to take them too late, but only you can decide. You will see that all the information directs you towards consulting qualified medical people before taking any medication. Be sure of all the 'medicinal compounds' before you administer them to yourself: they may not be 'efficacious in every case'.

Alternative Remedies.

Here we must proceed with caution. We are entering a corner shop of potential-herbalist-chemical-placebo belief, possibly akin to some form of witch doctoring or something that might be found in a Harry Potter story. I call it a 'shop' because many of the products are for sale and it is a case of 'buyer beware'. I'm not saying 'don't go there', but I am saying 'think carefully' and 'take care'. I am **not** endorsing anything that I may mention here.

Seasickness

Wristbands. The most frequently suggested alternative to drugs is to wear a bracelet or wristband that presses on the median nerve in the inside of the wrist about 35/40 mm above the hand. Explanations of the efficacy of this technique usually relate to acupuncture, at a point called P6. Get the point, or it might not work. The material that the solid bracelets are made from (often copper) can be offered as another alternative.

This is an area that can offer real commercial opportunities, so wristbands to *'reduce the **feeling** of nausea'* that *'doesn't act on*

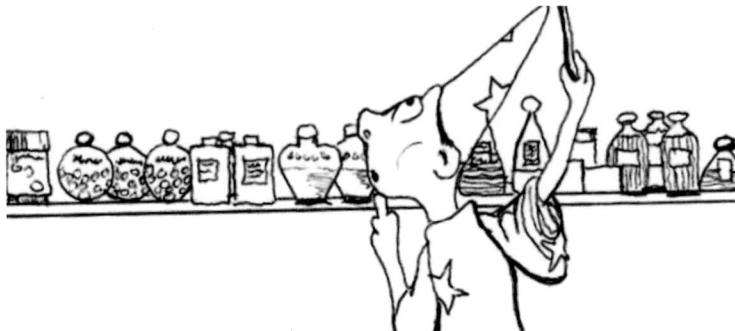

*the **causes** of nausea'* (wording in some adverts) can be offered at prices from £50 to £100+. They do this by delivering *'low-level electrical pulses'* to the skin and *'batteries are included'.* I have seen wristbands described as *'stylish'*, so you can make your own mind up about the mindset of those who produce and market them. You can decide whether they are for you. The elastic-band, pressure-pad types are cheaper, starting at £5+. They cost a bit more if they have a small magnet instead of a plastic button to apply the pressure. I got the feeling that a DIY solution, with additional benefits for the health of my wallet, was not beyond the limits of my ingenuity.

Aromatherapy. Much depends on individual preferences and beliefs. There is, perhaps, a 'food' link, with peppermint and ginger coming high on the list of preferred scents together with orange and lemon with the odd flower, such as geranium, thrown in. I wondered at the possibility of taking an actual orange or lemon aboard to ward off not only seasickness but also scurvy later in the voyage. (See also 'acids' in 'food later.)

More seriously, I have been told that on the (relatively short) sea crossing from the Italian mainland to the island of Capri, the crew give tourists fresh-cut slices of lemon to hold in their mouths. I was told that it seemed to work. I don't know whether it is the smell or the taste of the lemon that did the trick, but it may have been another effect, **distraction**.

If the mind is occupied with a simple activity it can damp down its concentration on other matters. I have seen this effect used as a temporary pain-relief measure, where gathering, then holding, moisture underneath the tongue and repeating a reassuring sentence three times didn't allow the pain to develop. I did not believe this could work until I tried it (to disprove it) and was surprised at its effectiveness. I thought that it worked, so the next time you hit your thumb with a hammer, give it a try (whilst nipping an ear lobe to dissipate pain messages being sent from the hand). My only logical explanation was that it 'distracted' the mind from registering the full effect of the pain. So could it be the same with the lemon slice? I have always wondered why dentists don't have a cartoon film running for their patients to watch whilst they are sitting in the chair. I think it would have a greater pain-relieving effect than staring at a blank ceiling. Patients aren't supposed to be laughing whilst they are in the chair, are they? Maybe the lemon works by aromatherapy? I have my doubts, but you can buy its bottled smell if you wish.

The one aroma to avoid (as already mentioned) is that of sickness itself, and a wondrous range of sick bags can be found for sale directly from the Internet or through chandlery catalogues. The choice covers several different styles, plastic-lined, biodegradable, fold-over tops or mouthpiece tops, to mention but a few. Along with these go disposable gloves, antibacterial wipes and pulped-paper sick bowls like those you find in hospital. I haven't seen this kind of equipment on any craft that I've been on, but perhaps they were all too small and the skippers too poor to include such kit.

Homeopathy. Here we return to the individual's attitude and strength of belief. When I read the 'contents' of some of these hugely diluted preparations I see that they can include what I think of as 'pseudo-scientific' words rather like the descriptive words used on hand cream lotions. Such lotions often have a main component called 'Aqua' (rather than 'Water'). So it is with homeopathy, where I have found 'Latinised' words like 'tabacum' and 'nux vomica' which instantly trigger word-links in the mind, unlike the word 'petroleum' (that was an ingredient), which seems straightforward enough (but foreign sounding enough?). Should you be swallowing these

29

potions? Not to worry; they are so diluted they won't have any 'side effects' according to those who market them. Now what do you make of that?

Sometimes you might be advised to apply potions behind your ears or spray them under your tongue.

It is sometimes difficult, but not impossible to logically link these products to everything else that is written here, but this does not mean to say that they do not work. It is up to individuals to test these and any other products for themselves if they wish.

If the wand-they-wave works for you ... use it!

Goggles. I cannot move on without a mention of the 'Anti Motion Seasickness Glasses' that I glimpsed in a chandlery catalogue.
They cost 'only £50' and look like a pair of swimming goggles with water inside the lenses. The blurb says that the fluid inside the frames creates a natural horizon so that your eyes send the same message to the brain as the inner ear. The claim for these specs is that they need only be worn for an average six minutes and that tests show them to be 95% effective. This seems to fall into the 'too

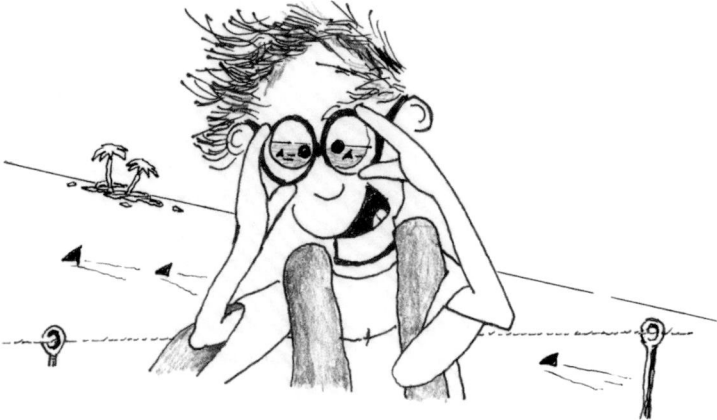

good to be true' category, but I have never tried them. Can you afford to, or should you use your own swimming goggles half-filled with water?

You can buy an audio CD, or ear plugs with valves to damp down air pressure in the inner ear. The experiments are all yours to try.

30

What to DO about seasickness on a yacht

Beginning the 'cure'.

(Well it's not really a 'cure', more an 'improvement')

Remember that **prevention** is better than cure.

Let us think of it more as a potential **Remedy**.

Food and energy

Much of what preceded this has related to the link between body and brain. It has been emphasised how hard the brain has to work, and this means that it needs more energy to keep up its higher work-rate. Medical books will tell you how a large proportion of the fuel that you take in is used to operate the brain. Allied to this, first aid books will explain how when the body is chilled, say, by falling into cold water a condition known as hypothermia will begin. Eventually, several stages later, this can lead to the brain not having sufficient energy to keep operating properly and it is possible that death can follow. We need not bother about this extreme here, but it is important to remember that food is the fuel, and if you don't have enough fuel being burned in the body, then that body will eventually begin to 'cool down' and, inevitably, slow down.

Most people are not aware of how this operates until they lose their food by being sick. Remember that it is commonplace to be sick several times and the sickness can go beyond the 'normal' sickness experienced onshore that is often caused by eating something that upsets the stomach. In such circumstances, once the offending material has been expelled, there is a good chance that the worst symptoms will subside and the sickness stop. This is not the case with seasickness. The movement that is causing the problem continues after you have been sick and so the body will be sick again even after all the food has gone. Many sufferers will bring up bile from the stomach and after that may still try to be sick, when there is nothing left to bring up. This is sometimes called 'dry retching'. At this point the body reacts by severe muscular contractions of the abdomen, which are exhausting, especially when the body is already weakened.

Seasickness

Internal cold

The sufferer will now be feeling cold and will be advised to wrap up well, to keep warm. The advice is good, but the effect is not what it should be. The body generates warmth inside by burning the fuel of food. Wrapping up is a process of adding insulation to stop this warmth from escaping and keeping the body warmer for longer. If there is no warmth being generated from within, then the insulating layers will feel to have only a limited effect. Yes, they are keeping in what little warmth there is, and they are also holding the cold conditions outside away from the body for longer, but they do not generate heat in themselves. It is possible to be well wrapped, but still be shivering under the layers, and this won't get better until more fuel is burned.

This is the problem:
**Putting more fuel in is the solution,
but eating makes you sick.**

First steps towards a remedy

A certain stage can be reached in sickness when time has passed without the sufferer being physically sick, yet they still feel nauseous. They are very cold and probably shivering. At this point they can swallow their own saliva without being sick. This is an odd thing to say. It shows how bad the sickness might have been. It might also be the first indicator that a certain stage of acceptance has been reached by the body. It is accepting a very small amount of liquid (that it has generated itself) down into the stomach and is not rejecting it. Can this situation be exploited? Taking in moisture to replace lost liquid to stave off dehydration is an important consideration.

If the sufferer can keep a few additional drops of water down for five or ten minutes without rejection they might be able to move to the next stage. The first step is to try to take the smallest amount of water possible and hold it in the mouth (warming it and effectively making it indistinguishable from saliva) before swallowing it. Will the body accept this? If it does not, then wait before trying again. If it does accept the water, then after a period of time try it again with a little more water. We are talking about small spoonfuls not mugfuls. A mug of cold water will almost certainly be rejected and the whole recovery process set back.

Seasickness

The aim of this tentative process is to gain acceptance from the stomach and eventually to begin to hold down some fuel (food). Often, the sufferer will not want to try food, because they just don't feel like it. The sickness sensation can be so similar to the feeling of being full and having a loss of appetite that they can be confused. It takes a conscious decision to overcome this deception of sensations and to try to 'eat' (it's not really 'eating') something. If the sufferer can succeed in adding the smallest amount of fuel to the liquid that is being accepted, then the true process of recovery can begin.

By sucking a few grains from a sweet, or dissolving just a sliver of a cheese biscuit or ginger biscuit (or whatever suits you) over a ten-minute span (see below) and keeping it down, you will begin to feel the miraculous effect of the warmth spreading through your body. It is amazing how small an amount of food can do this, but you must be patient and **not eat more** until you are sure that what you have eaten will not be rejected and your body is absorbing its beneficial effects. It must be held in the mouth and totally dissolved. It has to be **liquid only** by the time it is swallowed. You must be disciplined and patient. It is reward enough to stop the shivering. You must continue all the other actions of lying down and keeping your eyes closed. The **timing** of this is very difficult to judge, but it is the only answer to the problem of 'internal cold'. Only **energy** can cure that.

Energy remedy

Before you even get to this stage, you might have taken steps to help yourself. Your aim, right from the very beginning, should be to *conserve energy*. **Energy is the key.** It is needed to run your internal systems, especially the brain that needs to find the solutions and link the new networks. As far as it is humanly possible, right from the very start, as soon as you start to sail, you should try to follow a regime to restrict energy loss.

Never stand when you can sit.
Never sit when you can lie down.
Keep yourself warmly wrapped.

When lying down, wedge yourself in a position so you don't have to use muscles to restrict and control your body movement. On yachts this might mean not lying on your 'own' bunk, but on someone else's instead. This can be known as 'hot-bunking' as a relay of crew use the same secure bunk(s). It might mean not using a bunk, but lying on the floor instead. This can seem so unconventional to anyone who has not been on a boat before, that it is only undertaken with a feeling of embarrassment. Don't feel silly. If the floor is the best place and you are not in the way of everyone else, then lie on the floor. It is part of your 'cure', providing others know about it and don't fall over you in the dark. Being in the middle of the boat, low down, is where the movement is minimised. It is better than being at the ends, especially not at the bow where the movement and noise are the greatest

Removing protective sailing clothes takes a long time and a lot of energy. Much depends upon the conditions and the number of crew available, whether they are worn below deck. 'Full kit' can continue to be worn if you are lying on a resistant floor. Not removing all kit is often accepted on yachts especially in rough or challenging conditions if lying on seats and berths. This is rarely explained to newcomers. The basic rule is to try not to carry excessive salt water below. Take off wet jacket, harness, buoyancy, roll down oily trousers to boots, but keep trousers and boots on. Cover body with opened sleeping bag avoiding trousers/boots. This makes preparation to go on deck considerably easier and quicker, especially in the dark. Don't use strong light to get dressed. This cuts down on the visual information and preserves the night vision that will be needed.

Closing your eyes saves a great deal of brain processing energy (see *Snapshotting*, later). Deep breaths of fresh air help enormously once on deck, but there is a trade-off. Being down below in the cabin protects the face from the wind that constantly draws heat from the body when above deck.

Eating remedy

Allow me a disclaimer here.
I am only referring to people with normal health, as I have no knowledge of diabetes or any other individual health condition. Each person must see to their own safety, relating it to their own physical condition.

Before setting off you should have eaten a sufficient amount of food to keep you going, sufficiently long ago that it will be well digested and be supplying energy with not a huge amount of content remaining in the stomach to be lost in sickness. This should be the last major meal and it should consist of food that is easy to digest. All commentators agree that greasy or heavy foods should be avoided, as should excessive alcohol. Solid pieces of meat take a long time to digest. I have observed that some vegetable matter is often the slowest to be broken down. This may be open to discussion, but there is a standing joke about sickness that asks the question:

Why is it that you have always eaten carrots before being sick?

I must stress, this is advisory, for people in normal 'good health' only.

You should probably change your eating pattern.

A guide

It is better to eat very small amounts constantly than to eat major meals with long intervals in between.

The stomach seems better able to cope with a gentle, steady stream of food that is trickling energy into the system constantly.

It is easier to swallow soft, almost liquid content than to have to deal with large amounts of solid or very dry content. (Check the extract from *Serial Starship* and also John Mahon's advice under *The Complete Cure?* later.)

Gather a supply of suitable food and drink together before sailing, so that you don't have to go seeking it out. Experienced sailors fill flasks with hot drinks or soup in preparation for what is to come.

The best and most immediate form of energy is sugar

Food for energy. A bag of jelly babies (fruit jellies or wine gums) should be in a pocket that is safe from being dunked in seawater. They are predominantly sugar. You must NOT try to eat these all at once, but suck one or part of one very occasionally. They are no longer sweets; they are energy devices, more like pills to be taken at predetermined intervals as required to keep the body fuelled.

Food to settle the stomach. There is general agreement that ginger in all its forms comes top of the list. It has helped the

Seasickness

Chinese all these years and there are claims of a 'medicinal' effect in soothing the stomach. Some advice says to take it 12 to 24 hours before going to sea. Crystallised ginger will increase the sugar input and the woody residue can be chewed to maintain a steady flow of saliva. Maybe the residue should not be swallowed when exhausted? Dried fruit such as dried apricots will have a similar effect of giving something to chew on whilst also offering energy nourishment. Biscuits (ginger) or crisps (good for replenishing salt) crackers should be available, but they are not to be eaten in the conventional manner. Fragments should be placed in the mouth and dissolved there, slowly, prior to swallowing, possibly interspersed with 'dissected' jelly babies.

Having been sick, your initial mission is to **avoid eating solid foods**. You are attempting to extract the nutrients and energy they possess. Half a ginger biscuit in small pieces should take at least a quarter to half an hour to eat, and then there should be a break to give the stomach time to start absorbing it. If your stomach decides to reject it, the content will then be small.

If you have been sick, replacing the liquid is an important requirement, but you cannot just 'down' a whole glass of water. It has to be sipped very slowly, absorbed, just like the sugar sweets. Sweetened yoghurt could be useful. Fizzy drinks are to be avoided, but 'still' drinks with plenty of sugar should be considered. Part of the problem with an empty stomach is that the excess stomach acid has nothing to work upon. Try, therefore, to avoid strongly acidic drinks such as concentrated orange juice. However, I have experimented with sipping 'flat' Cola drinks and found them to be helpful. The calming effect is supposed to be from the phosphoric acid content and possibly the sugar, but the fizz probably doesn't help and neither does caffeine, so you have to work out for yourself what is best for you. Low-calorie drinks are, of course, useless for energy, but do supply liquid. The content of Energy drinks needs investigating by you. Drinks that are heavy on caffeine tend to make you urinate more and you are trying to retain moisture if you have been sick, so you have to strike the right balance. Alcohol dehydrates strongly.

Some people are helped by peppermint, so a tube or bag of mints should be good. Some 'energy' products such as Kendal Mint Cake are almost solid sugar with powerful mint flavouring.

Seasickness

Dealing with information-overload

Snapshotting remedy

Much emphasis has been placed on restricting visual information by keeping the eyes closed. This is VERY important. Keeping the eyes closed really helps, but it may seem difficult, even impossible to do as the sailor moves about in the boat down below. This is where 'snapshotting' comes in, using the well-known effect of 'persistence of vision'.

Look at the scene before you and then close your eyes. Out in the world that you have just been looking at everything is actually still there, and although you can't see it you can memorise the location of most things if you wish to. It's just that you don't usually bother too much about remembering things in this way. With eyes closed, you can reach out your hand and pick up anything of which you noted its position that is within arm's length. If you miss the object that you want, momentarily open your eyes (in the reverse of a blink) close them quickly and you will have a new picture, a snapshot of where the object actually is. Now you can reach it, pick it up and easily manipulate it, without actually looking. It is the same for longer distances, and you can try the technique when ashore in your own living room. Stand three or four paces from the light switch, 'snapshot' it and move to put your hand on it. You won't be very far off. If you are, just explore with the hand a bit. Or snapshot again.

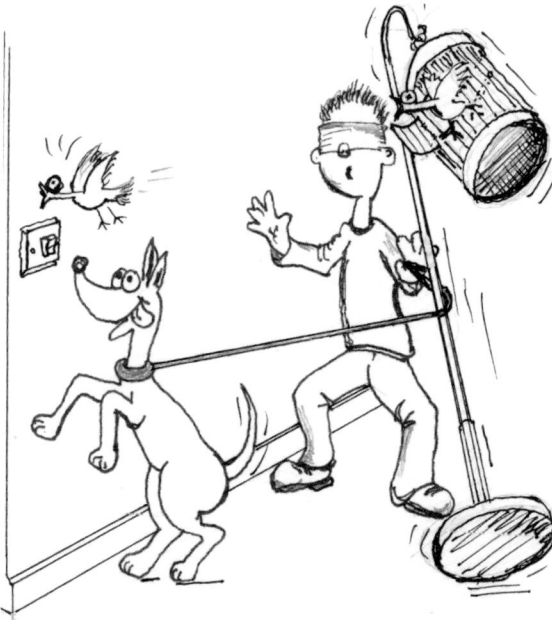

Seasickness

Okay, you have to be careful not to trip over the dog or knock over a vase of flowers, but you don't really need me to tell you that, do you? What is the practical use of this on board? It is going to save your brain a whole lot of 'visual blur' processing, a whole lot of information-overload.

For an 'advanced' example, the skipper and crew in the cockpit, beating to windward, may call down 'Make us three teas please.' You, the crew below, now have a complex task to perform involving lots of looking and judging ever-changing movements and locations in the cabin. This is exactly the kind of sick-making task, a bit like reading, that is likely to overload your systems. You know where everything is, but the visual processing might get you. Use snapshotting to get to the galley, to secure yourself and to assemble the components. Obviously the greatest dangers are in lighting a stove or securing and manipulating boiling water, and for something like this you can look constantly; but half a dozen snapshots can cover a huge part of the process. (*Incidentally, wedge the cups in the sink or in a bowl when it comes to pouring the liquids and don't fill them too full.*) You will avoid much of the visual mental processing that could bring on sickness symptoms.

Sea legs and positive thinking

Lying wedged in, with your eyes closed, well wrapped, but not sweating, occasionally sucking a mint, fruit jelly or crisp is about the best that you can do, in seasickness avoidance, working towards the remedy. Doing this may be delaying any decision that the brain might make to force you take these very actions, simply because you are doing them already. The longer the brain gets to reassess and retrain for the circumstances the better.

You can also try clearly thinking or even saying out loud (quietly to yourself so as not to scare the rest of the crew) *I am on a boat. This is just the movement of the boat. I like the gentle rocking. Nothing to worry about. It is just the boat that moves like this. I'll soon get used to it.*

Now I can't prove that this will have any effect other than to make you feel a bit foolish, but it is the positive attitude and messages that the brain needs. Its value is probably in overriding negative thoughts. Remember that 'thoughts and emotions' have the power to trigger seasickness. Some people will say it helps and others will say that it makes no difference, but you can try it if you want.

Seasickness

Keeping up this positive mantra can push negative thoughts to the back of your mind. It is the 'distraction' effect mentioned earlier, and you may find yourself nodding off to sleep in the process. This would be very good. This provides rest for the muscles and the space that the brain needs to readjust.

Once it has done that, you will begin to get your sea legs and you should start to come out of the other side of the difficulty. Getting your sea legs is the process whereby the brain is re-educated so that it realises that it doesn't have to respond to every small movement, that doorway sides need not necessarily be upright and that it can tune down its responses, yet still cover the essential running of the body systems.

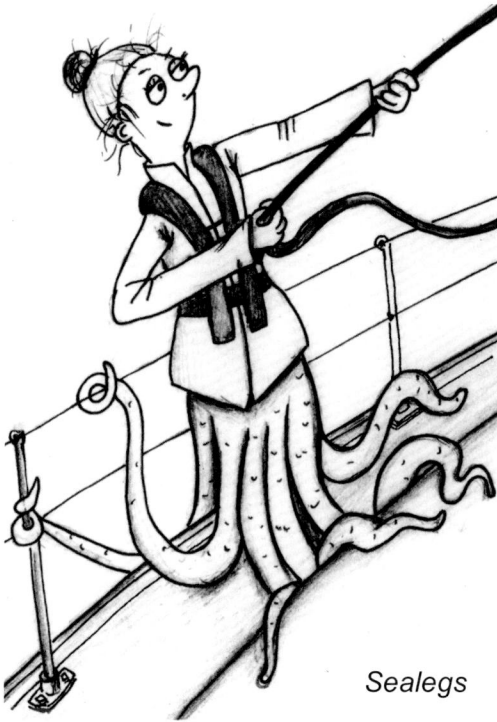

Sealegs

Your '*sealegs*' will need a readjustment when you eventually return to land. You may have seen on news reports, some long-distance sailors being supported as they step ashore and stagger slightly at the unyielding solidity of the land. Yachtsmen become accustomed to a sensation of 'lightness' or 'floating' if they sit or lie still in a warm dim environment ashore. The first time of lying in bed away from the boat can produce a feeling of your legs floating upwards that is all part of the retuning process to get your '*landlegs*' back again. It is quite an enjoyable sensation if you just let yourself, literally, float along with it.

39

Some ways of operating on boats at sea

Including some sailing mistakes

The very best start to a sailing journey would be to acclimatise on the boat before setting off. The boat could be anchored away from the still water of a marina so that it can turn in response to wind and tide whilst lifting and falling to wave and swell. This almost never happens. Most yachts have a journey to make, and often it is 'the sooner the better', and the inexperienced crew just has to go along with what is happening around them.

The most common mistake for the novice crew to make when embarking on a yachting journey is to stay in the cockpit for too long. There is interest and activity in casting off and motoring down the harbour. There is much scenery to be admired and other craft to see. The bustle of raising sail, setting the course and watching the receding land whilst discussing everything with the other members of the crew, is what sailing is all about. There is a great deal to see and absorb and this takes up brain space, but new crew are not aware of that. The watches should soon be set if the journey is to be extended, and it is then that those without immediate responsibility for the boat should go into their 'energy conservation' mode, but in the excitement of the newness of things they most often don't.

Staying on deck at this point and not saving energy is where the real problems slowly begin. Depending on sea state, an hour later newcomers on deck may begin to feel 'queasy'. Skippers will generally advise going below to keep warm, but the queasy crew now need the deep breaths of fresh air to keep them going. Looking below at the swaying cabin, they know they probably won't make it.

They don't know the 'process' of being sick on a yacht. What should you do if you are down below? Can you use the toilet? (*Yes.*) Can you use the sink? (*Not good, the plughole is too small, but better than the floor.*) Should they rush up on deck? (*Possible, cockpit floor from standing inside companionway is acceptable, where it can be washed down and has big drains.*) What will happen if they don't make it? They might have had a briefing on safety harnesses, man overboard, fire extinguishers and the watch system, but nobody has said anything about being sick. They feel naïve about asking. Nobody else is talking about it. Shouldn't everybody have a bowl allocated? They begin to appreciate just how long it is going to take to remove their sailing clothes. Dare they risk it? Sitting still and looking out at the horizon, the one true, trustworthy indicator of what is horizontal (and therefore what is upright) whilst taking deep breaths, is the limit of their ability, so they stay.

Someone will suggest trying to go on the helm a bit as this improves things, and **it does,** but it increases the energy drain on muscles and energy requirement of the brain dramatically. It allows good reference to the horizon, in relationship to the boat movement and that helps, but essentially the novice sailor is heading into an energy cul-de-sac. When they come off the helm, they still will not want to go below, they know for certain that they cannot eat or drink anything and so they are trapped in the cold environment on deck. They are usually sick, somewhere at about this point if they haven't been sick earlier and then they are locked on deck as the most convenient place to be sick is overboard, to leeward.

Now comes the cycle of how to get warm without wanting to eat and without going below? Any movement is energy-sapping and taking off full sailing kit including boots, harness and lifejacket is exhausting. It will take anything up to half an hour to dress or undress fully in a small yacht in anything of a seaway. The best hope now for breaking the cycle comes from sleep to allow the brain to recover and energy to be restored. Nightfall also greatly reduces the amount of visual input. Darkness naturally restricts what the eyes can take in and the demand upon the brain is greatly reduced, allowing it to adjust more rapidly to the new situation. Being in the dark helps a great deal.

The best introduction to sailing a yacht at sea, for the novice sailor, is that they join in and see the departure. They then go below, keep warm and get some rest by falling asleep. They begin to eat and drink small amounts constantly. They use snapshotting when down below to restrict visual input, and when they come back on deck to help run the ship it is approaching darkness, which has a similar effect. They have the right food and drink with them.

Onboard regime

The way that yachts are run usually depends upon the skipper. It is in the skipper's best interest to have crew that are all fit enough to stand their watches. In this way everybody gets their full rest time,

41

as more rest is needed than when ashore, especially when working watches around the clock. Most landlubbers are not accustomed to getting up and working at two or three o'clock in the morning, outside in the cold and rain. A skipper of any worth should try to support the crew over the first series of watches until the worst of the seasickness is over and each person can contribute positively to the running of the boat. One way to do this is for the skipper not to be in the initial watch rota (depending on numbers available). She/He has many additional duties and responsibilities, particularly concerned with navigation, communication and the safety of the boat, but if the skipper is not in the rota they can have the flexibility to assist the crew to find their sea legs.

It is counter-productive to force a badly sick crewperson on deck for a full watch just because the whole watch timings for the next three days have already been written down before departure. Flexibility is the word for the first 24+ hours, and a good skipper should know the strengths and weaknesses of themselves and the crew and be prepared to shorten a watch or extend it with agreement, or stand in themselves, as necessary, in order to get 'ill' people well again, as soon as possible.

The continuing remedy

The first steps are the critical ones. Anyone who can consume and hold down a biscuit or a couple of sweets is on the way up. It is then up to them to monitor themselves and to think of what they can eat and when, keeping the earlier advisory 'rules' for food in mind. If they have a watch coming up they must not get caught out halfway through it without access to sufficient food and drink to keep them going and replace the energy and liquid that they are using up. As soon as their watch is finished they must return to snapshotting and energy conservation as they go below without delay to make their way to their secure sleeping area. Gradually they will know whether they have cracked the problem as they eat more and begin to feel so much better. Getting back to a consistent, varied diet is important. All this eating sugar, biscuits and crisps can then be relegated if conditions remain steady and appetite returns. Soup, bread, toast, tinned fruit, dried fruit, canned rice pudding etc. can then begin to creep onto the menu.

The complete 'Cure'?

I don't know if there is one. I have always thought that if the conditions at sea get bad enough, then anybody can be seasick. That goes for ordinary mortals like you and me. Yes, I can be sick and have been sick when I got scared enough and tired enough. Why else would I have thought about all this stuff? There are some Supermen and Wonder-women out there, of course, but I'm talking about ordinary folk.

This is an extract from *Serial Starship* first published in *Multihull International* magazine, taking only those sections that relate to the seasickness situation, mainly of fear and fatigue. This was aboard a 35ft. boat at this point sailing from Land's End to Milford Haven when it was caught out in the open Atlantic in what was recorded as storm force 10, with all crew aboard being seasick. No modern electronic navigation systems were on board.

'My thoughts were not clearly ordered, but mixed with the lurch of the boat, the blue of the sky, the majesty of the elements in full force, bracing myself for the next wave, and the overwhelming sound of it all. I watched the boat, getting a feel of her speed, how accurately we held the compass course, roughly how much leeway we were making. The helmsman looked across with the smallest flicker of a smile and nodded his head. It was about midday.

I tried to consider our situation from the point of view of navigation. The conventional sitting at a table with ruler and dividers was totally impossible. The smallest glance at a chart brought an overwhelming retching and further exhaustion. Even the less conventional methods of just laying objects across the chart to get a rough idea of direction were only slightly feasible at times, but very difficult to execute. There was a mass of mental calculations, all very simple of course when you are sitting at home or in the classroom, but it was a major mental effort to calculate how many hours from 7.30 to 2.45pm and then multiply by knots to find out how far we had travelled. Were we doing four knots or six? It made an incredible difference. Exactly how far was our journey? It spanned three different charts with different scales. The lethargy of total exhaustion made such calculations seem like 'Mastermind' questions. Outwardly I appeared to be almost in a coma, but inwardly I wrestled to keep our track. I did not have the energy for conversation, but John helped by double-checking for me. I'd mumble 'How far is Land's End to Padstow?' as he scanned the chart, and ten minutes later as we passed each other he'd give me a figure. He'd wearily ask 'What do you think about speed?' and ten minutes later I'd give him my estimate. Together in this way we reached a consensus of position in our own minds. I forced myself to study, be sick, study, be sick, ignoring the discomfort until I had sorted out a confirmation based on our agreed figures. In a case such as this it wasn't possible to have pinpoint accuracy, but it was possible to have an outline strategy, and I was feeling generally satisfied with our progress because in spite of everything, I felt that we were falling within the best course of action given our difficult starting point and the extreme discomfort that we were undergoing.

Our course had been determined by the safest approach to the wave faces. The tide would now be taking us westwards and we needed to counteract this if we were not to miss Wales altogether. In mid afternoon I asked for a course of 030m and we managed to hold this slightly more reaching course without extreme danger in the wave pattern.

At about four in the afternoon Jerry suddenly recovered from being laid low, and I finally managed to make a little food stay inside me. I had been sucking sweets slowly, which usually effects a cure as the sugar gives me energy, but on this occasion it just didn't seem to work. I noticed John trying cheese crackers, and fortunately it did the trick for me also. It was quite remarkable what effect just four crackers had. Almost immediately I stopped feeling quite so cold, and started to feel much more positive. Jerry too coming fresher to the scene seemed positive and optimistic. Next he noticed that there were seabirds about, and this was a significant observation. Since leaving the land behind us we had seen only those isolated seabirds, which seemingly glide right under the falling wave crests, storm birds soaring, banking, and feeding right into the jaws of hell, but the birds that we saw now were different.'

Here we see various factors that we have outlined being combined in the text:
- The tiring effect of bracing against movement
- The reading activity directly precipitating sickness
- Tiredness affecting the ability to calculate
- The need to have a strategy
- The curative effect of eating
- Finding the right things to eat
- Allowing the crew time to recover and become useful again
- The value of positive thinking

Seasickness

Getting control by **understanding** all the elements of what happens and taking the appropriate actions to minimise the adverse effects is what this has been about. People want to know how long it will take, and I can only say that it depends upon the individual, the journey, the boat, the personnel, the weather and most of all the sea. Anyone at sea in any craft is only there because the sea and weather conditions are allowing it to happen. Many people can control seasickness after a couple of days, some three, four, or five. A short sea journey of only a day or so is no real test of whether a person can overcome mal-de-mer because it would probably involve a long time being sick, without the counterbalancing reward of enjoying sailing once the difficulties have been overcome.

Finding out how other people have been affected by seasickness and what they did about it, such as in the passage above, is quite difficult. In most sailing stories the account will just say that the people concerned were sick, but then continue, sometimes without further comment or at most, say that they recovered after a couple of days. One notable exception to this is John Mahon in his autobiography '*Drink Up and Be a Man*', published by Seafarer Books, where seasickness is mentioned as early as the second line in the book. This is a unique and engrossing account of life 'below decks' (*rather than 'stairs'*) as a steward aboard the classic liners in their heyday and on commercial vessels. It is a 'warts and all' story with plain speaking. John's first real 'taste' of the problem came on a ferry in the 1960s travelling from his native Ireland to England on the Dublin – Holyhead ferry. Having used this route myself relatively recently I can say that quality and standards have now changed. In the old days facilities were 'basic'. I have extracted only the words relating to seasickness from this passage of events. This is what John writes:

'Someone near me started retching, and that was enough to send me scurrying to the toilet to puke. I found the place crowded with men and boys of all ages in various forms of disarray. The smell of body odour mingled with vomit and the sight of it all over the sinks and on the floor caused me to be violently sick, and when the ordeal was over I gingerly stepped out of that stinking place and found it hard to keep my balance with the movement of the ship. One moment I was walking up a steep hill and the next I was holding onto the rail with all my strength to prevent myself from being thrown forward.

Seasickness

An elderly steward came along the alleyway and saw my plight. 'Give me your arm, lad, I'll help you. There's an empty cabin just around the corner where you can get your head down. You look all in.'

He led me to the dimly lit twin berth cabin. 'You lie down now and I'll be back with something to settle your stomach.' I contemplated giving him a tip when he returned with a packet of cream crackers. 'You probably don't want to eat anything,' he said, 'and you're thinking you'll never want to eat anything again, but believe me, if you can just get a couple of these biscuits down, you'll feel much better. They'll help to dry up the acid in your stomach. I'll be back to see you later, try to get a bit of sleep.'

I ate two biscuits and lay as still as I could, and the next thing I knew the steward was back and the movement of the ship was less erratic. 'We're out of the worst of it now,' he said. 'How do you feel?'

'Much better thank you,' I replied.

'Where are you heading for?' he asked.

'London for a job on the big passenger liners. I have three years hotel experience and I think I'll stick to that because of the way that I've been feeling on this trip.'

'That's rubbish you're talking. Don't worry about the way you're feeling now, this can be one of the roughest sea passages in the world.' He told me that on his first trip to sea he had been employed as a scullion and every time he looked at a plate with even a bit of food on it he was sick, and it was worse when he had nothing to bring up, and that's when he was introduced to dry toast and cream crackers. He was sick on and off for about a week and then he never looked back.'

Several other points that have made at various places within this book can be seen in operation in this short extract:
* The sickness being precipitated by others being affected
* Lying down
* The dimly lit cabin
* Eating when not wanting to
* The choice of food (to settle the stomach)
* Sleeping
* The likelihood of recovery
* The ability to work whilst being sick

Seasickness

On this last point, John as a steward serving food frequently had to advise the liner's passengers on dealing with their own seasickness, and he continues to recommend the method that he had learned.

'We briefly discussed the menu and how the movement of the vessel was affecting all the family (passengers he was serving). None of them could face a cooked breakfast, but they felt that they should eat something. I suggested cereals with just a small amount of milk, or better still without milk, and maybe some fresh dry toast. They settled for tea and toast only. Easy for me, and thankfully, as I was feeling queasy myself.'

With his vast experience he continues to use this advice to this day.

What are your alternatives to trying such methods?

Armed with the appropriate knowledge you can now try for symptom control yourself, but as I said at the beginning, there is no guarantee of total success. There is no single magic bullet. What are your alternatives other than to try this system? Well, you can just resign yourself to the position in which you find yourself and be sick until it stops.

Tough?

You could also take the traditional 'tough' attitude of one skipper I once knew, who advocated, *'Drink seawater, be a man, and be sick. That's the way we did it when I was a lad.'* I have to mention that this chap didn't drink seawater. He was sick. At times, he couldn't be roused from his bunk to stand his watches. He remained unaware of who helmed his boat during the night and when eventually he came on watch feeling queasy he would cut it to a minimum, handing over early to novice crew that he knew to be inexperienced and seasick, thus extending his own time off watch. He didn't only do this once.

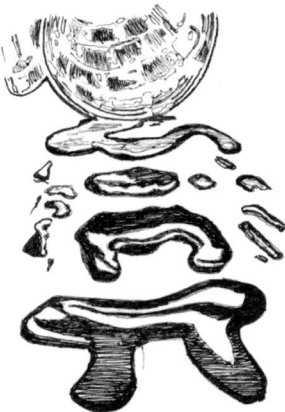

Seasickness

I leave it to you to decide whether this kind of advice is for the benefit of the sufferer, or whether it is to perpetuate a 'traditional', uncomfortable initiation once popular amongst a certain brand of physical male 'worker'. It comes from an age of poverty and hardship where *'the sooner tha's sick an 'as done wi' it, the sooner tha' kin get back te shovellin' coal, (*or *scrubbin t'-deck) the better'.* Or whatever the task of grinding toil was that they were engaged in at the time, hauling halliards, gutting fish, turning capstans. In those days they didn't have time for 'mother's boys' with soft hands. They didn't carry passengers. You either worked or you got off. This was fine, then, but the method probably has limited viability on modern leisure yachts where volunteer crew step aboard for the pleasure of learning more about sailing. However, having said this, if you think this is the solution for you, don't let me stand in your way.

Try it. *'It'll do thee gudd!'*

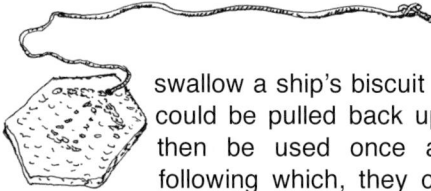

Even more medieval is another tale of having to swallow a ship's biscuit on a piece of string, so that it could be pulled back up to precipitate sickness and then be used once again on the next sufferer, following which, they could be sent back up again onto the yardarm. There was no doctor's sick-note and no delay with these methods. The words 'kill or cure' come to mind.

I can only say that I hope that you are more fortunate and get a skipper with an approach to the problem of seasickness based on patient understanding rather than on pressing ignorance.

It is worth including a brief extract from a best-selling, Victorian book *Letters from High Latitudes*, published by The Merlin Press (now Seafarer Books) relating to Arctic sailing in 1856. Shortly after departure the doctor was sea sick and it was decided to *'observe the phenomena of seasickness from a scientific point of view. The doctor set to work most conscientiously to discover some remedy. Brandy, prussic acid, opium, champagne, ginger, mutton-chops, and tumblers of salt water, were successively exhibited; but regretfully after a few minutes, each in turn re-exhibited itself with monotonous punctuality. Indeed it was thought at one time that he would never get over it.'* He did of course. Mixing opium with champagne did not work then. It will not work now. Do not try it.

Be positive

If you like sailing, remember, the illness phase is part of the training period for the body. Something wonderful is happening. The architecture of your brain is starting to change, to build a new neural network. It is putting in place the capacity to deal with this unusual set of circumstances. This restructuring is called plasticity. The more urgent the need, the faster the brain will do this, and being sick has moved the requirement to construct the new systems into the 'emergency' category. This is a wondrous ability of your unconscious mind, but you have to be patient. Your body cannot learn instantly, all training takes **time**. The brain has to make the adjustments and have known strategies to access, suited to the seagoing situation, only then will your vulnerability diminish.

If you can get through the uncomfortable stages for the first time, there is every hope that next time the body's adaptation will be that much more rapid. If you can build up your experience, you can achieve a situation where you could go to sea expecting *not* to be sick. Who knows, eventually it could be you cooking the bacon and egg on the first night out, but please, spare a thought for the novices on board.

Good luck. I am wishing that this 'cure by understanding' is for you and you won't always have to 'sit under a tree'.

I sincerely hope so.